D1135075

FENG SHUI

Making Your Space Sacred

SADIE MAE

**Andrews McMeel
Publishing**

Kansas City

Design by Amy Ray

ISBN: 0-7407-2330-8

CONTENTS

Introduction

Feng Shui (FUNG SHWAY) is the ancient Chinese art of finding balance and peace in your surroundings. Feng Shui literally means "wind and water."

In Ancient China, it was believed that for the luck of the living to be good, the ancestors' gravesites had to be protected from both wind and water.

The essentials of Feng Shui grew out of this belief. Its principles have been observed in the East for many centuries. By incorporating a few hints from Feng Shui into your life, you can make changes to your home that will bring more health and greater happiness to those you love.

Origins

In ancient China, the natural world was studied devoutly. The concepts that developed are the basis of Feng Shui. Understanding these concepts—the energy of Ch'i, and the balancing of Yin and Yang—is very important to creating good Feng Shui.

Ch'i is the life energy that pervades everything. When Ch'i is flowing abundantly in your home, the results are health, happiness, and good fortune.

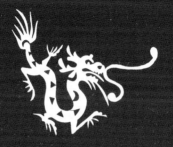

The Chinese consider the green
dragon to be a symbol of life.
The breath of the dragon is
another way of describing Ch'i.

Yin and Yang are the two complementary forces that are present in all of life. Like night and day, they exist together. Yin is feminine and Yang is masculine. A perfect balance of Yin and Yang in your home creates harmony and well being. An imbalance will make you feel uncomfortable.

YIN	YANG
Water	Fire
Soft	Hard
Quiet	Loud
Still	Active
Closed	Open
Dark	Light

The mythical origins of Feng Shui lay deep in the history of China. A story is told of a man named Fu Xi who was searching for the secrets of life. Fu Xi was convinced that everything was governed by one universal law and he devoted his life to discovering the secret.

One day as Fu Xi was meditating by the Li river, a dragon leapt out of the water. Fu Xi noticed that the dragon had strange markings on its back and he drew them in the sand in order to study them.

Gradually Fu Xi began to realize that these markings were the clue he had been looking for. From them he devised the eight trigrams, which contain the secrets of all the various cycles of life, and of changes that take place in nature and in the human spirit. These trigrams are used in Feng Shui to describe the different aspects that contribute to a happy home.

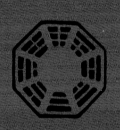

Over many centuries the eight trigrams were combined to form the Pa Kua, a compass that can be placed over a home or room to help determine the most beneficial placement of objects. Each direction of the Pa Kua is identified with a life aspiration.

A further development in Feng Shui was made in China during a flood of the legendary River Lo. The people were told that in order for the flood waters to recede, a sacrifice to the river god was needed. Each time one was made, a turtle emerged from the river and circled the sacrifice, indicating its inadequacy.

Trying to figure out what to do, the Emperor of China was standing on the banks of the river. As he looked down at his feet, he saw the divine turtle with magical markings upon his back.

Adding up the numbers of these markings in many different ways, the emperor arrived each time with the number fifteen. Applying this magic number to the sacrifice, the river god was appeased, and the flood waters abated.

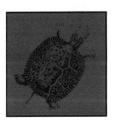

The magic markings that the Emperor Yu-Huang had seen upon the turtle's back were combined with the trigrams of the Pa Kua to make the Lo Shu grid, which is used to determine the optimum relationship of all the elements that make a home. The numbers are used to calculate everything from spatial dimensions to auspicious periods of time for various activities.

4	9	2
3	5	7
8	1	6

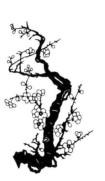

Feng Shui Tips

A bowl of fruit on the
kitchen or dining room
table signifies
abundance.

It creates positive
energy and enhances
prosperity.

Keep both your
refrigerator
and your pantry
well stocked.
A sparse pantry or
refrigerator indicates
a lack of abundance.

When pouring a cup of
tea for a guest, do not
point the spout toward
your visitor.

The spout sends out
hostile energy which
can create
misunderstanding.

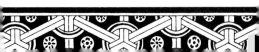

Dining chairs should be
even in number.

Even numbers
represent luck, and
odd numbers
represent loneliness.

When positioning your bed, ensure that the foot of the bed does not point directly toward the door. Energy enters rapidly through your feet and this may cause sleepless nights. If you can't move the bed, close the door.

Do not have your bed
directly under a
window, as this
encourages you to
listen all night for
intruders and prevents
you from sleeping.

Make sure that your
bedroom is bathed in
light. Dimly lit rooms
bring gloom and
sluggish energy.

The electromagnetic
fields from a television
are a serious disruption
to energy. If you must
keep a TV in the
bedroom, keep it in a
cabinet or cover it with
a cloth so that the
screen is not visible
when you sleep.

Allow sufficient room
under the bed for Ch'i
to flow. Empty space
under your bed will
make you feel lighter
and more carefree.

To improve your love
life, bring some
yellow into the
bedroom. It will aid
communication.

Refrain from hanging
items on the backs of
doors. Doing this
increases the weight of
the door and adds more
struggle to your life.

Keep windows clean to
ensure clarity of vision
in your life.

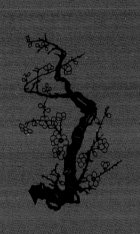

If you widen the front
path to your house,
it will make
coming home
more inviting.

Do not place furniture
directly below
exposed beams.
This could result in
severe headaches,
bad luck,
and business problems.

Rounded objects create harmony in the home, whereas sharp corners create disruptive energy. Keep this in mind when furnishing your home.

Comfort is key
in cultivating the
positive flow of Ch'i.

Make certain that
the furniture in all the
rooms of your house
is relaxing and
comfortable.

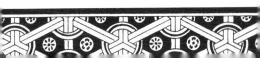

Select antique or
second hand
furniture carefully.
It may have bad
Ch'i from a
previous owner.

Red will
intensify passion.
It is a lucky color, and
is associated with fire,
happiness, and
warmth.

Use light green and
blue to create a calm,
soothing energy.

Blue is also the
color of protection.
Calm and peaceful, it
encourages inspiration.

Warm colors such as
terra-cotta and
yellow enhance
positive feelings and
encourage a
heartfelt approach
to life.

White enhances
creativity.

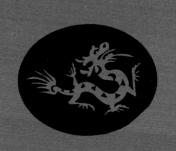

Gold will attract
brightness and
great honor.

Fluorescent lighting
contains negative ions.
Avoid using it.

Table and floor lamps
create comfortable
pools of light that can
be used to illuminate
dark areas and
encourage more Ch'i
into any areas that
need activating.
Like your life, a
room needs light.

Keep your mirrors
clean. Dust and dirt
reduce the effectiveness
of mirrors.

The reflection you
see in a mirror is
what other people
see in you.

Mirrors reflect Ch'i
and create
liveliness. They can
be very useful in
awkward places and
can be used
to create space.

A Pa Kua mirror can
be placed on the
outside of your house
to deflect harmful Ch'i.

Do not hang the Pa
Kua mirror indoors.
Its intensity will
confuse things.

Hanging a mirror
opposite a door will
inhibit the flow of Ch'i
into the room. This
encourages undue
confrontation, and may
alienate you.

Mirrors in your dining
room symbolically
double the amount
of food on the table.
This creates a feeling
of well-being that will
benefit you, your family,
and your guests.

Mirrors should be
framed unless they are
recessed. Raw edges
on a mirror
will produce raw edges
in your life.

Cracked mirrors should
be removed from your
house, as they
fragment your life.

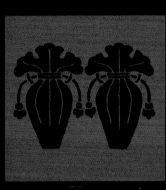

When positioning
mirrors, do not place
them to reflect each
other. Energy will
bounce around and go
nowhere.

Use still-life drawings
to bring calm to your
home and active art
to create more
movement.

Ancient coins can be
used as a decoration to
stimulate wealth.

When hanging on a
wall, the Chinese
character for double
happiness will
strengthen and enhance
your relationship.

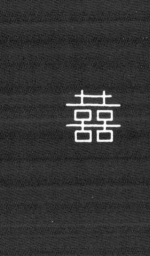

Wind chimes placed
where air moves will
make music, enliven
the space, and
encourage Ch'i.

Wind chimes are useful
for remedying
background noises,
such as air-conditioning
units or the refrigerator.

Water, particularly
moving water, attracts
Ch'i and money.

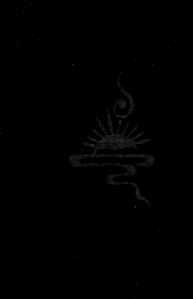

Waterfalls or fountains by the entrance to your home encourage a flow of positive energy. It is essential that the water is always clean and flows continuously.

Check that there are no
leaking faucets in your
home. They indicate
money flowing away
from you.

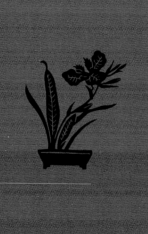

A vase or bowl of fresh flowers in your living room will create positive energy and make your family and guests feel more cheerful.

Do not place cacti or
other plants with thorns
indoors as they give out
bad energy and may
cause arguments.

When used outdoors,
however, they will help
protect your home
from harm.

A live plant can
stimulate the energy of
a bedroom. However,
do not have too many
plants in this room
as they can use up all
the available Ch'i.

Placing plants near
your computer
equipment will help to
absorb the harmful
energies being emitted.

Upward-shooting,
round-leafed indoor
plants increase the
oxygen level and lift the
energy in a room.

Birds and fish make
wonderful pets.
They both
symbolize
wealth.

Household pets
can be very
helpful in activating
good Feng Shui as
they are always
moving from
room to room,
encouraging energy
to flow.

Do not keep ashes
of a beloved pet
inside your house.
This represents death.

Keep your pets in the
back portion of your
house. This keeps the
front available for
people and positive
Ch'i to enter
without difficulty.

Summary

The art of Feng Shui has been practiced for centuries. Those who become familiar with its principles use them in their homes, their businesses, and in their gardens. Feng Shui can be applied to any building structure or landscape situation. Its affects are always beneficial.

There are those who consider Feng Shui to be a fine science, with principles that can be learned. Like all art—and like life—Feng Shui is best practiced by those who are willing to delve deeply into it, who experiment with its many aspects.

The rules of Feng Shui cannot be learned by rote, for the truest expressions of balance and harmony must be felt to be understood. The information in this small book is but a place to begin a wonderful journey of discovery and an ever deepening relationship with the world in which you live.